Sound Sleep, Smart Wake Up

Turn Your Bed Into: Mat

DAVE MCALLEN

DEDICATION

To Rose Williams, my mentor in sport.

CONTENTS

Household Items

Conclusion

ACKNOWLEDGMENTS

Thank you to all my readers and users of my manuals and handbooks. I especially value your honest feedback.

INTRODUCTION

You are not ill, you are only tired, so tired, it gives you something to worry about: Why am I so tired?

Or, you can't sleep. You always lay there in bed, but at dawn, you can relate all the things that happened in the neighborhood during the night. When you heard the alarm each morning, you wish that from heaven, some powerful voice shout at the belligerent thing with a thunderous "shut that thing off!"

You are not alone when it

comes to the matter of tiredness. Many people are often tired and they can't sleep. Most people under today's world hectic pace return home from anywhere, tired. They go to bed tired, hoping to wake up refreshed. Still, when they are awake in the morning, and they are tired.

Many of us however no longer feel fatigued. We sleep soundly and wake up smartly. What's the secret? This book in your hand is robust with it.

Rest assured that we are not advertising some drugs, vitamins or some food supplements here. In fact, what you will learn from this handbook will show you how never to get tired again and spare you of the risk of depending on drugs to manage fatigue.

WHAT IS TIREDNESS OR FATIGUE?

"The state of wishing for sleep or rest." (Lexico, based on Oxford) The same source defines fatigue as "Extreme tiredness resulting from mental or physical exertion or illness."

WHY WE GET TIRED

As already underlined in the introduction, there's no longer any dumb wonder about why we get tired easily these days. Keeping with the fast pace of our world today is hectic. We all feel tired often, after every engaging day. Night sleep is no longer enough to refresh us. And alarm clocks now cause our hearts to skip beats morning by morning.

A NEW THREAT?

In the pre-industrial age, people were easily fatigued because human effort was needed to overcome virtually all the jobs needed for human existence. The situation often required that people of that history exerted themselves over long hours doing manual labours. Such labours included lifting of heavy loads that overtax their muscles and joints. They also had to put in static efforts when the job to be done made such demands upon them. This means that their muscles would have to keep parts of the body in a fixed position. That time, most works were done in uncomfortable positions.

At that point in history, there was high rate of fatigue. Illnesses with symptoms that fall under the group of Repetitive Strain Injury (RSI) were common too.

THE FALL AND RISE OF FATIGUE

In the nineteenth century when the inventions of industrial machines came to relieve manual labour, the rate of tiredness and fatigue fell.

But as history moves deeper into modernism, the old threat return and even worse. There's high rate of chronic stress, inflammation of the spine, lumbago, headaches, insomnia, CVA risk, etc. Even works that people do and would not get fatigued early in the industrial age, can now wear workers out in our century. You may wonder: what has changed?

Before our generation, man was the master of the newly developed machines. Man told the machines what to do for him. He was in perfect control. But as history travels, there was tremendous improvements to our machines which gradually grow them from being our slaves to our masters. Today, the machines tell us what to do, when to do them and how to do them. We thus become the slaves. A machine may instruct you to move your hands in a particular way, how many times and for how long it wants the movements.

Thus we have no control over the job we do. We have no choice but to accept jobs that damage our health.

This condition is not limited to the workstation. At home, our domestic machines also dictate what we have to do. For example, our television tells us to glue our eyes to the screen, thereby forcing our muscles to keep some parts of our bodies static. This is a contributing factor to getting tired at home. Use of mobile devices is another good example of domestic machine instructions that overtax the ligaments and tendons etc, especially those of our upper limbs.

THE ANALYSIS OF FATIGUE

Keep in mind that not one, but a group of effects are responsible for your fatigue. All the factors in this group, affect the muscles, the joints, the spine, the lower back, tendons, ligaments, etc., mentioned above. In its advanced stage, tiredness can produce discomfort and pains that may prevent sleep.

However, many mental health experts believe that causes of fatigue are not limited to effects on physical body parts. The relationship between your mental faculty and work or home environment is involved. The work you do, your worker-management experiences, the work climate itself, your level of involvement and the routine nature of what you do are strongly linked to the factors responsible for getting tiredness from work.

Similar conditions are cited for getting domestic fatigued apart from the effects on the physical body members. What you do as a wife, your husband-wife relationship, the parents-children connection, and the home atmosphere are among the mental causes underlined.

Other medical experts highlight the amount of control you have over the way the home or the workplace is organized. For example, because of modern technology, the workplace dictates for the worker as said before, what to do, when and how to do it. These forms of arrangements have led to workers losing all the control over his job. He works almost instinctively, oblivious of positions that can cause discomfort, such as sitting awkwardly, in a static effort, etc. At home, it is the same downside of technology. You may be quite engrossed with your mobile, PC or TV, etc, without realizing that you are bent-sitting.

HOW SERIOUS IS THE MATTER?

Untreated tiredness can develop into chronic stress or chronic fatigue. Repetitive Strain Injury (RSI) can also result. In some advanced cases, untreated RSI can cause deformity.

The chances of recovery from fatigue is much greater if you pay attention to it in the early stages.

POPULAR RECOMMENDATIONS FOR BATTLING TIREDNESS

Before we unveil our incredible cure, it is necessary to look at some popular recommendations for preventing tiredness. Many experts favour ergonomics. This is a field of applied science that deals with arrangement of things in ways that people and things interact most efficiently and securely.

This means that time, efforts and funds must be invested to make man and his workplace blend with each other. Tools should be improved. A worker's mental and emotional needs should be tabled and the data should be used to his advantage. But don't let your employer do all the changes of the workplace for you. Play the biggest part. Pour out before him what your tastes are on tools and your workstation itself. You wear the shoes, so, you know better where they ache your feet. If you work hard to improve your work climate, you will escape most of the factors responsible for getting tired and fatigued.

Another suggestion is adoption of a work calendar that provides for recess or changes that rotates different types of jobs among the workers. This is especially important in the case of prevention of RSI.

REVEALING OUR INCREDIBLE CURE

As you have the patience to read this handbook to this point, we need to congratulate you. You are now about to unveil the secret to overcoming tiredness.

Drugs violate our system. We use them when there's nothing else to do. The techniques you will learn will greatly reduce your use of them. Even some pains from forms of fatigues, he RSI, don't respond to medicine.

What do you need? Just small weights, your bed or

any flat surface, such as a mat, a long table or a bench. Once you have these materials ready, you are all set. What types of weights do you need?

We recommend the sack weight. Sack weight is safe as it contains no small parts that can cause injuries when it fell. In addition, it is incapable of damaging the floor indoors or other things it may meet if it slips accidentally.

The weight is clean and will not pose some hygiene risks as it is used indoors. The outer materials are usually velvet or Jean. So, it can be used on the bed and anywhere in the house. Later, we will guide you through the process of making them economically at home.

HOW TO USE THEM

Have a drink of water. Then, stretch out on the bed and take a small weight with each of your hands.

Keep your legs straight. Your head and shoulders should not rest on the bed. Keep them hanging down at the edge of the bed. Your lower back should be on the bed to keep the weight from sliding you down. Keep the hands together. Then, very slowly, stretch them over your head until they are in the same straight line with the rest of your straightened body.

Slowly bring them back to your legs while still keeping them straight with the weights in them. Repeat the process as many times as you can. Pause regularly to take a slow deep breath in and out.

There are no hard and fast rules as to how many times you lift or how heavy the weights must be. It has to do with what "YOU" can take. And you will enjoy the activity as you feel the good effect all over your body.

Now separate the hands and stretch one to a direction. Do the same thing with the other hand. Extend the hand to other directions, one hand, then, the other - North, south, east, west, northeast, northwest, nothsouth, and on and on. In fact, your hands need to take the weight through more than trajectory routes.

Smaller weights are better to achieve this objective. That means, you need weight pairs of different sizes at your disposal.

You will realize that some pressure is exerted on certain parts of your body with every direction your hand goes. Continue, trying to cover a wide-ranging area you can think of.

Put your hands together sometimes with the weights in them, and suspend them a little above your knees. Then, keep raising them up, down with very slight movements until you feel pains in the muscles of the hands, your abdomen and around your spine. Pause awhile to breathe in and out.

Now you still lay on your back in bed. Lift the hands. Keep them together with the weights still gripped with them. Extend them straight over your head (not over your face). Move them slightly up, down, up, down, with very slight movements until you feel pains in certain parts of your body including the neck and your chest.

You can also attach small weights to your legs. Use these with caution. Make sure the ones you use here are very small as you take the pelvis into consideration.

Stretch out straight on a flat surface. Then, try to lift the legs but slowly, up, down, up, down. There's no rule as to how high or low the legs go. Just raise and drop them, but make sure they are kept straight. Breathe in and out deeply.

When you stand up, you can also take the weights with you. Hold them together and throw your hands with them to each of your sides, one after the other. You can be changing postures. Stand at ease, at attention, bend from your waist, or stand straight. It may not be necessary to keep your hands straight at this time. Your posture as you twist will determine how you will keep them. For effective results, your legs shouldn't move from their positions. Hang the hands down or raise them to any level you want. You can bend and keep adjusting the level and keep twisting. Breathe in and out deeply as you twist.

There are other very effective ways to use these weights. Sit on the floor, place one weight on your neck and twist. You can put a light one there and try to put your forehead to your knees. Breathe in and out deeply.

You can also place a weight on you neck and squat until your lower buttocks touch your heels. Spend a few seconds there. Then stand straight. Repeat the process again and again. Take a deep breath, in and out.

On your own, you can discern the specific muscles that you use most and strengthen them. Stronger muscles will help you to perform the necessary tasks at work without getting tired.

When you stand, you will feel as if some operations have been performed upon your body and some pounds of flesh were removed from there. You feel very light. Have another drink of water and then, take a long shower.

WHEN TO USE THE SACK WEIGHTS

"When you wake up, imitate your dog or cat. Notice how your pet stretches its muscles before getting on with a new day. Do the same. And, while you're at it, repeat those stretches a few times during the day. This is essential for keeping your bones and muscles healthy." (g98 12/22 pp. 16-19) So, if you have access to the weights throughout the day, use them a few times during the day. Start when you wake up. Conclude when you prepare to sleep.

SIDE-EFFECTS

Beginners feel sharp pains in some parts of their bodies. This is due to the force exerted upon some participating tissues to overcome the friction in them. This has pulled them beyond their range of movement.

If you have this experience, do not panic. All you have to do is not to try to stretch yourself beyond what you can bear at the beginning. In fact, as you will see, you don't need to be under stress to get the most out of this form of exercise.

You need to enjoy yourself when using the sack weight. If you are not careful, you will sleep off while exercising. Just stop and then move the hands and the legs in varied directions. Bring them back again. Continue to repeat the process until your nerves and muscles are free enough not to pain you.

It could take days for some, and a few weeks for the bodies of other people to gain flexibility.

THE QUESTION OF BODYBUILDING

This question is there too. Many people don't like bodybuilding. So, are you afraid that using the sack weighs will increase your shoulder muscles and give Six Packs to your belly? That is nothing to worry about.

First, you need to reckon that the weight we mean here are small, something that is just enough to make a difference to your normal body weight. What you need to stretch your muscles and relax your nerves won't increase your arbs.

Second, we do not recommend any size of weight you will need. We leave that to your judgement. Whatever size of weight you are deciding on, however, should take your normal body weight into cognizance. The larger your body weight, the bigger the size of the weight that may affect it efficiently.

That is why it is beneficial if weights of different sizes are available. When you are tired, it may be difficult to exercise with a heavy weight. So, when you have the pairs in a number of sizes, you will be able to use what is convenient for you at a given time.

BENEFITS

The heart is the centre of life in our body. So, our first area of interest is the heart. These activities with the sack weights will strengthen the heart muscles. A healthy heart pumps better, which will increase the amount of oxygen available for our muscles to do their work. Such a healthy heart is also likely to function for a long time to prolong our lives.

Drinking of water before and after the activities helps to prevent stroke, CVA.

Such water intake expands your blood volume and the activities accelerate the circulation from the heart with ease. So, oxygen-carrying blood is present in all parts of your body, including all the areas of the brain.

Use of sack weights strengthens other core muscles of your body – the muscles of the heart, the kidneys, the liver, the pancreas, the back and the abdomen.

They are strongly recommended for the reviving of the breast support muscles in women.

Orthopedic doctors often cite this series of activities as a correctional measure for postural defects, improvement of bone density and muscle relaxant.

NOTE: If you ever had a surgery, find out from your

doctor if you can use small weights for fitness. He can advise you, whether the activities that require exertion is safe for you.

OTHER CORRECTED PROBLEMS

The following are some of the ailments in the list that small weights can correct. Backaches, obesity, enlargement of the liver, bulging stomach, stress, sleeplessness, some kidney issues, repetitive strain injury, RSI, waist pains, burning legs, headaches, high and low blood pressure, normal tears formation, and stomach regulation.

MADE ECONOMICALLY FROM CHEAP HOUSEHOLD ITEMS

Get some tough fabric materials. We usually recommend Jeans or Velvet. Cut them in the shapes as shown in the succeeding page:

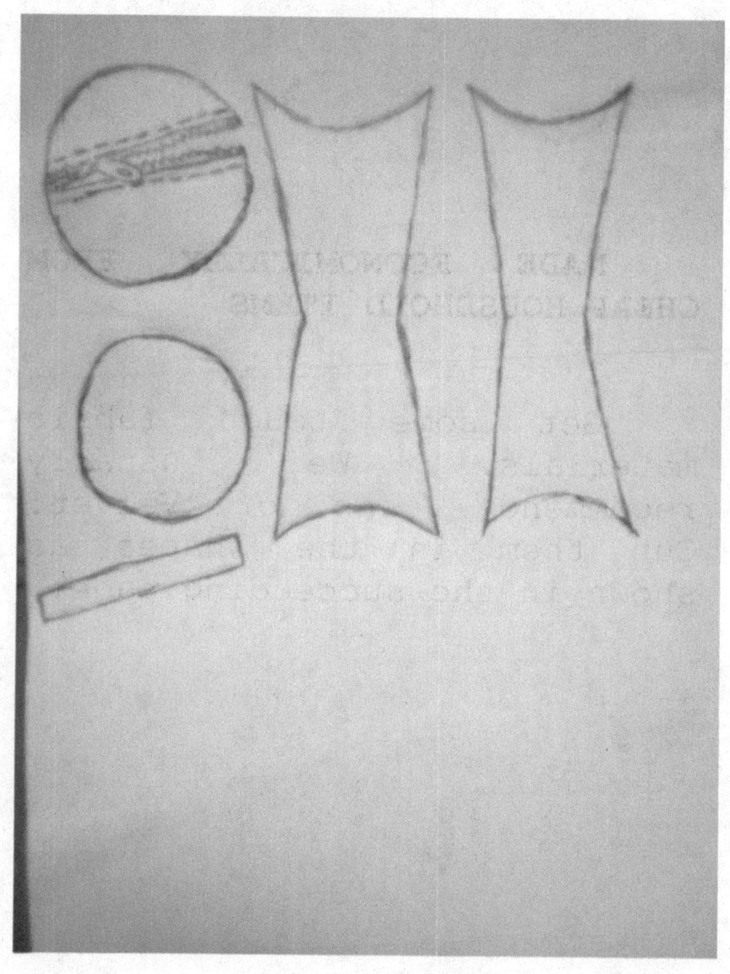

Let your tailor help you to join the twin shape pieces. He should turn the back of the material and sew. The result is an open-ended pipe-like club.

Next, he should cover the openings with the two circle pieces, one on each side. You noticed that a zip is sewn to the middle of one of the circled pieces. Your tailor will then sew the last piece, a narrow flap, over the zipper to hide it from view.

Further, he will turn the inside out so that the front of the material is what is in view. Then, get a polyethylene sack that is longer and wider than the cloth sack. Gently raise the flap, pull the zipper to open and insert the polyethylene sack into the cloth sack, letting some surplus of the polyethylene to come out over the mouth of the cloth sack.

Get some fine sand and load it into the sack, through the mouth of the polyethylene bag. Shake as you fill. Continue to load until the sack can no longer bend.

Next, tie the mouth of the polyethylene bag and force it back into the cloth sack. Finally pull the zipper over the head of the polyethylene to close the sack. Then, let the flap cover the zip from view. Now, you have completed all the processes of making the sack weight. Make more in the same way until you have a number of pairs in different sizes.

You can now begins to use your weights.

As the weights begin to get soiled, put them in water and wash. The purpose of the polyethylene bag in the sack is to keep the sand from getting wet when the weights are washed.

CONCLUSION

The benefits of using these small sack weights may prove greater than the time it costs. And you might never be tired again.

APPRECIATION

    Thanks for reading this book. Please, give me a little more of your time and leave me a review.

    Thank you, Dave McAllen, Author.